I0411352

WHY DO WE NEED FOOD?

Understanding how our body uses food and how it affects each one of us

Marianne Duvall

ISBN-13: 978-1489532022
ISBN-10: 1489532021

Contents

Introduction

We are surrounded by information, guidance and even government direction about what food we should and shouldn't eat.

Walk into any bookshop and you'll see that one area that has put on more and more weight over recent years, are the bookshelves carrying all the books on diet, nutrition and how to lose weight – especially how to lose weight. The diet industry is massive.

But we seem to be more confused than ever about food and what we should eat for good health.

The phrase 'we are what we eat', trips easily off the tongue, but they are often just words, not taken seriously or even understood.

But it is absolutely true.

Archaeologists can tell from ancient bones whether people in a prehistoric settlement were getting their protein from meat or fish – we literally are what we eat.

Nowadays we have lost all connection with what our food actually is and where it comes from. For most people it comes from the supermarket or the fast food outlet. We take more care about what fuel we put into our cars than we do about the fuel we try to run our own bodies on.

Understanding that the food we put in our mouths is literally the fuel we are powered with, is the first step to improving our diet and our health. Understanding what that fuel is, how we should create the premium mix of fuel in our own kitchens and how that fuel works, is vital in the process of improving general health and helping avoid chronic illnesses such as heart disease, diabetes and cancer.

Learning what food is

Governments have tried to help educate the general population about food in various different ways over the years.

In the United States of America they came up with a very visual approach to good nutrition – the Food Guide Pyramid.

It was introduced in 2005 by the United States Department of Agriculture (USDA) and the United States Department of Health and Human Services (HHS) to help the general public understand how to create a balanced diet from a good range of foods.

It is a simple, visual interpretation of a healthy life style, giving basic messages about healthy eating and physical activity, which apply to everyone - the steps in the diagram represent physical activity and the coloured bands of the pyramid represent the different food groups.

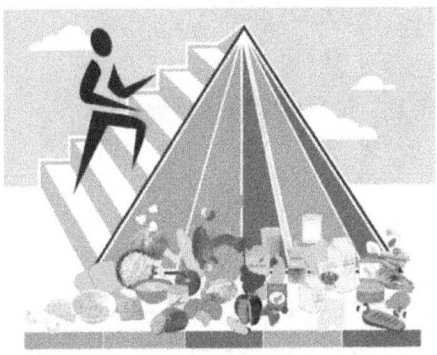

It divides food into types represented by six colour bands:

Grains, vegetables, fruit, milk, meat & beans and oils

The Pyramid shape shows the greater value of foods with little or no added sugar or solid fat at the bottom of the pyramid, rising to the narrower sections representing less healthy choices at top.

Recently they replaced the food pyramid with the food plate, a visual and easy to understand guide to balancing the food types on your plate.

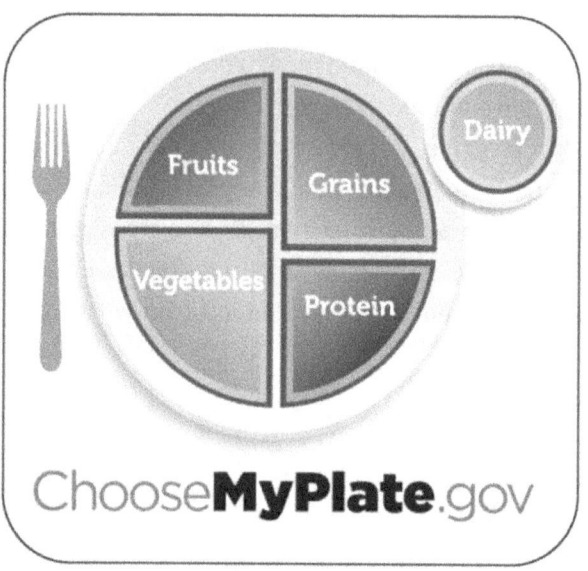

There are other visual guides available, but the aim of all of them is to actually show what a healthy balance of food groups actually is, but they don't explain why you need a mix of food groups or what each food group will do for you. And unfortunately they don't give much guidance on how much of each food group you should put on your plate, and portion size has increased a huge amount over recent years!

Portion Size

20 or 30 years ago you would bake dainty fairy cakes for a party, now you bake muffins or cup cakes for almost any occasion, or even worse, you go to the local shops and buy them, so that you don't even know what the ingredients are. Not only do we eat them more often, they are far larger and smothered with cream and icing. This is being repeated in all types of food choices. We are encouraged to super-size our meals.

A slice of cake with your coffee is huge nowadays in comparison with a few years ago and some coffee cups could be used as flower pots! And then there's the coffee. We're no longer satisfied with a simple coffee, it has to be latte, mocha, macchiato, cappuccino, mocha latte – the list seems endless and so does the calorie count.

We're encouraged to 'super size' or choose a 'king-size' serving, soft drink cups resemble buckets and we're tempted with all you can eat buffets, extra large servings and endless refills of soda. Even the plates have put on weight! A standard dinner plate that you buy today is much larger than one you would have bought twenty years ago.

As a general guide, a portion of fruit or vegetables is about what you can hold in your hand – this means that you make allowances for the fact that people are different sizes and a delicate five foot woman doesn't need as much food as a six foot five man- a wonderful example of nature creating its own guidelines for us.

Most of the information about portion sizes does have to be based on an average adult, who is aiming to maintain an existing healthy weight, so do remember to take this into account when you are adapting the advice to suit you or other members of your family.

The general guideline is to have 8 to 10 portions of starchy or grain food, three portions of meat, fish or other proteins, three portions of dairy foods and at least five portions of fruit or vegetables.

Again, taking into account your size, a portion of starchy or grain food would be about one slice of bread, half a baked potato, three tablespoons of boiled pasta, half a scone, three small crackers or three tablespoons of breakfast cereal. So in practice, you might have nine tablespoons of breakfast cereal (three portions), two slices of bread to make a sandwich (two portions) and six tablespoons of rice (three portions) to make up your curry in the evening.

Three portions of protein could be made up of two medium-sized eggs (one portion), 100 g of raw lean meat (one portion) and five tablespoons of baked beans, which is about half a standard tin (one portion). For vegetarians, four tablespoons of lentils or chick peas is about one portion, and a small handful of nuts would also be a portion.

Three portions of dairy food could be made up from a small glass of milk (one portion), a small pot of yoghurt (one portion), about 30 g of cheese, which is about the size of a matchbox (one portion) or about two tablespoons of cottage cheese.

Fruit and vegetables should make up the main part of your diet and you should have at least five portions a day, but remember that many fruits include a lot of natural sugar, so making up your five portions from grapes, strawberries, blueberries, melon and pineapple may be very healthy from a vitamin point of view, but not quite so good from the point of view of restricting your sugars, even if they are natural. This is particularly important for anyone living with diabetes.

A portion of fruit or vegetable is approximately 80 g, but a good guideline is the amount that can fit in your hand, for instance, a small apple, about 10 grapes or about three heaped tablespoons of peas or carrots. A small glass of fruit juice is also a portion, but only one a day counts towards your 5 a day.

Although the UK recommends '5 a day', other countries have different advice. The USA recommends 9 a day, Australia, 5 portions of vegetables plus two of fruit while Greece goes for six servings of vegetables and three of fruit. So really, the five a day guideline in a minimum to aim for, and of course it should be part of your healthy diet rather than just adding five more pieces of fruit to a diet that is already too heavy in calories!

It's also important to remember that potatoes don't count as one of your 5 a day - although sweet potatoes do – so a portion of fries every day isn't what they are recommending!

Is Good nutrition boring?

Many people see healthy eating as boring.

That in order to be healthy you have to cut out all the tasty food and treats, ban burgers, crush chips, delete delicious cakes!

The problem with this idea is that as soon as something is banned, it becomes the one thing you fixate on - the one thing you suddenly can't do without and instead of having a single biscuit you deny yourself any biscuits at all and then give in and eat a whole packet!

The whole denial idea is one of the main reasons for the huge failure rate of dieting. No other industry could survive with that kind of failure rate – but of course in a diet, it's always 'your fault' when you fail. Of course it isn't! It's the fault of the endlessly restrictive diet plans, most of which have nothing to do with healthy eating.

Healthy eating is nothing to do with a lifetime of denial, it is about understanding food and learning how to balance your diet. It's also about learning how to enjoy the food and how to take back control of your mealtimes and your food choices from the food manufacturers, fast-food chains and supermarkets.

So, once you understand the basics of good diet and nutrition and the fact that it isn't about banning foods, it is important to make sure that you have variety in your food choices.

Planning ahead and preparing menus may seem tedious and lacking in spontaneity, but in fact it can help increase variety in your meals and it saves time. It's far too easy to reach for the same old idea day after day if you have to make a choice when you're hungry - cheese sandwich again!

Planning ahead helps you choose a variety of fruit and vegetables as well as helping you to be organised with healthy versions of bread and cereals.

Using colour is an excellent way of making food look more interesting and of creating different combinations of nutrients. Red peppers and tomatoes, oranges and carrots, spring greens and spinach, blackcurrants and aubergine - when you start looking, the fruit and veg aisles at the supermarket are like a painter's pallet and mixing the colours in your food is an excellent way in ensuring that you get a good combination of vitamins and minerals.

How much food should we eat?

Before planning meals, it's important to know what fuel and how much of it we actually need.

The amount of food, the calories we need to consume, varies according to gender, weight and lifestyle, although the percentages of each type of food remain more constant. Someone very active or very involved in physical sport will require a greater percentage of protein in the dietary mix than someone more sedentary, while someone with diabetes will need a lower percentage of carbohydrates than average.

We have become used to the idea that burning calories is something that we do when we exercise – which of course we do, but that's certainly not the whole story.

When we eat we take energy in, and actually living uses up energy, the difference between the two is the energy balance. So if you eat the same amount of energy as you use, the weight will remain the same, if you eat more energy than you use you will gain weight and if you eat less than you use, you will lose weight.

We have been almost brainwashed into thinking that we only use calories when we exercise and therefore that almost all of food you take in is too much unless we spend the rest of the time running around the block or visiting the gym.

But in fact there are three different areas that make up the total energy consumed by the body - to get scientific for a moment - they are the Basal Metabolic Rate (BMR), the energy used in physical activity and the thermic effect of food.

Understanding that our body uses energy - and the term calorie is just a measure of energy - simply by existing, can help break the guilt link that the diet industry has created, which can make us all think that every calorie we put into our mouth should be burnt off in some form of organised exercise.

That is the dangerous idea behind starvation diets that limit the calorie intake to 300 or 400 cal a day. Of course you will lose weight; you are not taking in the number of calories that your body uses in basic survival. But that is also the reason that you will put the weight back on once you start eating again, your body cannot survive without food and choosing to go without food will put your body into starvation mode, altering your metabolism and affecting how you will process food in the long-term.

The BMR (basal metabolic rate) is the energy we use in the basic functions of living, so the measurement is for the body at rest. It does vary for each individual but a guideline is approximately 1.1kcal per minute for an adult. Muscle uses more energy which means that in general men have a higher BMR than women and younger people have more muscle than older people and so have a higher BMR, although children have a higher BMR in proportion to their size because rapid growth requires energy. The BMR is approximately 75% of your energy requirements.

Of course we also burn energy in physical activity, although physical activity doesn't just mean running on the treadmill it means moving! As a general guide, 20 - 30% of the body's total energy use is through physical activity, although it does vary with the intensity of activity. On average, walking would use approximately 100 kcal per 30 minutes while running would use about three times as much.

One of the important things about exercise is we not only use energy while actually exercising, the body continues to work more efficiently even after the exercise has stopped.

The third type of energy used is the thermal effect of food (TEF) - eating and processing food uses some of the energy that is provided by the food. This calculation is quite simple, the TEF = the total calories consumed x 10%, so 2000 calories a day x 0.10 = 200 kcal in TEF.

You don't need to work out these calculations, it just helpful to know that we do actually use and need food and the calories it contains, for normal everyday living.

What is a healthy weight?

There are plenty of charts that will give weight ranges for different heights, but a good guide is the Body Mass Index (BMI). This is your weight in kilograms, divided by your height in metres squared. You can find a number of tools online which will help you work out your BMI if you want to.

The BMI is an alternative way to check that your weight falls into the acceptable range, although it is important to remember that it is not a direct measurement of body fat. It is worked out using weight, which includes fat and muscle. An individual, who is very fit, such as an athlete, will have extra muscle which may tip them over the normal BMI range.

Understanding what calories are, how your body uses them and what weight range is healthy for your size and lifestyle, is an important guideline to being able to understand food and nutrition and how it will affect you.

We have relied on the food industry to tell us what is good and bad for far too long and we have lost in knowledge that we really need to be able to understand what we are eating what we should be eating and what effect it has on us in the long-term. This loss of knowledge has gone hand-in-hand with an ever-increasing problem with obesity and chronic illnesses such as diabetes and heart disease.

It's time to take control back and to understand what our food choices are what types of food we should have and in what proportions and how our food choices can improve our health and lifestyle.

Why do we need the different food groups?

Any nutritional guide, such as the food pyramid or food plate, gives a guideline for how much we need from each of the food groups and food labelling will show how much comes from carbohydrates, protein and fats. But apart from knowing what type of food is from what group, what do they actually do?

Although there are diets that suggest you should completely cut out a food group – some suggest you should cut out carbohydrates altogether, others cut out fat while some people try to eliminate salt. Some people struggle to get protein in their diet – especially vegetarians or vegans who cut out animal produce from their diet without replacing the protein properly. People who are trying to control cholesterol can also end up restricting their protein intake.

But the fact is that our bodies have developed over hundreds of thousands of years to work on a balanced diet, and although many of our modern food technology and modern eating habits have interfered with the natural patterns of food, we still need a good balance of food groups, in the right overall quantities for good health.

As a general guide your daily diet should be made up of approximately

33% bread, cereals and potatoes

33% fruit and vegetables

17% proteins – meat, fish, beans, nuts

17% milk & diary

8% fats & sugars.

The different foods also supply the different minerals and vitamins that we need for good health.

Again, we seem to have developed an idea that vitamins and minerals come in pills in little bottles – or sometimes quite big bottles! The food that we consume should give us the vitamins and minerals that we need.

The main exception to this is Vitamin D. The main source of this vital vitamin is the reaction of the skin to sunlight. Ideally you should have sunlight on your forearms for about 20minutes a day to produce enough Vitamin D. This isn't always easy! We work indoors more, don't always have great weather and many people either cover up or never leave the house without being coated in sun protection, so Vitamin D deficiency is a growing problem and in this case supplements can be the answer, even being prescribed by doctors.

The minerals we need come directly from food, we cannot produce them in the body. They come through the food chain from the plants that grow in the soils that contain the minerals. This can lead to a general deficiency in some minerals when the crops are grown in an area of the world devoid of certain minerals but you should be able to get the mix that you need by having a mix of food stuffs grown in different parts of the world and in different soils.

What are carbohydrates?

Carbohydrates are the basis of a healthy diet as long as we choose the right ones. They are obtained from grains, rice, pasta, bread, vegetables, fruit, pulses and dairy products. They not only supply the body with the glucose it needs, they are also a source of vitamins, minerals and dietary fibre. Unfortunately a packet of crisps or a biscuit, while still being carbohydrates, don't add much more than empty calories to the diet.

Why do we need carbohydrate?

Carbohydrates are sugar compounds. Life is fuelled by the sun and plants get their energy directly from the sun, growing when they are exposed to light. Although we need sunlight ourselves (to produce vitamin D) we can't directly convert the energy of the sun to power our bodies, so we get it from the plants.

Once we've eaten them, carbohydrates are broken down into glucose in the body, which is the fuel our brains require to function. Carbohydrates also fuel other vital functions in the body and provide the main source of fuel for physical activity.

The body can only store a limited amount of carbohydrate, which is why it is important to eat regularly, especially for an active lifestyle. However, excess carbohydrates are stored by the body as fat.

If you restrict your carbohydrate intake to less than your body requires to function, it will rely on the glucose that has been stored in fatty tissue as glycogen, in effect burning up the body's own protein tissue – that is muscle. If this goes on for long enough, eventually the body will run out of fuel and die. In the short term, that is why a restricted carbohydrate diet such as the protein reliant Atkins Diet, will result in weight loss. But you should remember that it's not only the fat around your tummy that is storing the glycogen, your muscles are where you get your strength to move, and the heart is a muscle as well.

Carbohydrate also helps in calcium absorption, the digestion of food by providing the nutrients for the friendly bacteria in the intestinal tract, helps lower cholesterol and regulates blood pressure.

Not all carbohydrates are the same.

Carbohydrates come in three varieties: Simple carbohydrates, Complex carbohydrates and dietary fibre. Dietary fibre cannot provide the body with energy, as the digestive system in unable to break it down into the usable sugars, but it is important to the health of the digestive system in helping to remove waste from the body.

Simple carbohydrates contain one or two units of sugar, complex carbohydrates contain more than two units connected together.

Simple carbohydrates are basically – simple! Their sugar structure can be broken down in to glucose very fast by the body once we eat them, which means that they are processed through the digestion very fast, can be turned into stored energy – fat – very fast and the energy that they provide is also gone very fast. So when we talk about needing a sugar fix, we mean exactly that – a quick, nutritionally useless, quick surge of energy that will leave us feel hungry and tired and in need of another sugar fix.

Foods such as highly processed white bread, sweets, cakes, biscuits, soda, fruit juice, chocolate, mashed potatoes, milk or processed cereals all fall into this bracket. So you can see that a breakfast of highly processed cereal with sugar and milk, a slice of white toast with jam and a glass of fruit juice will leave you reaching for a donut and soda by mid morning!

Complex carbohydrates are – more complex! They take longer to be broken down into glucose in the body, your system has to work harder for its energy, which means that it isn't crying out for more food within a couple of hours.

Wholemeal bread and cereal are complex carbohydrates, your body has to digest the outer shell of the grain to get to the energy inside it. Vegetables are also in this bracket, as are beans and lentils.

Knowing the difference between these types of carbohydrate can make a very big difference to how healthy your diet is. Choosing highly refined white bread instead of a wholegrain loaf can mean that you are hungrier faster and much more likely to reach for a snack to keep you going.

What is the Glycemic Index?

The important factor in choosing carbohydrates for your diet is how fast the body can break down the food into glucose. The Glycemic Index (GI) has been developed to measure how fast a food is digested and turned into glucose. Foods are ranked from 0 to 100 based on this speed.

A food with a high GI – 70 or more, will break down rapidly and give your body fast energy. This is important if you need to replace energy fast, for instance after strenuous exercise, or for a diabetic suffering a hypoglycaemic attack. However it is not good in general as the body will use up the energy supplied by the food quickly and you will be hungry again.

Foods with a medium GI – 56-69, will release their glucose more slowly, while those with a low GI – 55 or less, will take the longest to digest and will result in a much slower rise in blood sugar. Therefore, choosing low GI varieties such as wholegrain bread rather than white bread and brown rice rather than risotto rice will mean that your body takes longer to digest the food and you will avoid the sugar spikes and lows than can make you reach for snacks soon after a meal.

Many foods, including a large number of brands on the supermarket shelves, have been tested and there are books that will provide lists of the GI of different foods. As a general guide, the more processed a food, the higher the GI. You should choose food varieties that have to be processed inside the body rather than in a factory, choose whole grains and brown rice rather than fine ground French bread and risotto.

What is the Glycemic Load?

The GI gives the measurement of individual carbohydrate foods, and the GL of a food depends on the amount of carbohydrate in a serving. This means that a large amount of a low GI food can still cause a spike in blood glucose. Of course, we also eat meals that are a combination of foods. The Glycemic Load (GL), derived by Professor Willet from the Harvard Medical School, is a more accurate way of judging the rise in blood glucose. It gives a good estimate of the quality (GI) but also the quantity of carbohydrate in a portion of food.

To work out the GL of a food you multiply its GI by the amount of carbohydrate per portion and divide by 100. One unit of GL has approximately the same affect as 1 gram of glucose.

This means that in real terms some low GI foods have quite a high GL because of how much carbohydrate there is in a normal portion, while some high GI foods have a much lower GL because a normal portion has a low amount of carbohydrate.

Beetroot has a high GI – after all a lot of refined sugar is made from sugar beet. But you would have to eat a huge amount of beetroot to get that much carbohydrate, so it is a low GL food.

If you would like to know more about the GI and GL systems, there are many books and websites to look at. Although it is often sold as just another fad diet idea, choosing your food and meal plans from this system should be seen as a plan for a long term healthy lifestyle and it can be particularly beneficial in treating diabetes or poly-cystic ovarian syndrome, where insulin resistance is a serious problem and can lead to long term health problems caused by too much glucose in the blood.

Why do we need protein?

Protein can be used as a fuel for the body if there isn't sufficient carbohydrate to meet all energy needs, when this happens amino acids from the protein are converted into glucose.

But the real purpose of protein is for growth and development as well as regulating bodily functions. Every cell and tissue in the body contains protein – muscle tissue, bone, tendons, internal organs, hair, skin and even nails, and although the body can convert protein into carbohydrate if needed, it can't convert carbohydrate into protein.

Meat, poultry, fish, eggs, dairy products such as milk, yoghurt and cheese are all very good forms of protein providing the amino acids that the body needs, although they also contain fats, especially saturated fat. Plant forms of protein such as nuts, pulses, seeds and grains also provide protein but must be combined with other foods, because on their own, they don't contain the full range of amino acids.

A meal of baked beans on wholegrain toast is a very healthy mix of plant proteins.

The food industry has also developed a number of alternatives to meat protein in recent years in response to the demand for vegetarian and low fat alternatives to meat.

Soya based alternatives such as bean curd and miso are used traditionally in the Far East but are now popular in the west as well. Soya can also be processed into texturised vegetable protein such as soya mince, which can then be used as a meat replacement in recipes for those who want to avoid meat.

You can also find a range of meals featuring Mycoprotein which is sold commercially as 'Quorn®' and is an alternative source of protein extracted from a special variety of fungus

Protein is essential for good health, it helps maintain fluid balance in the tissues, carry oxygen, transport nutrients in and out of the cells and regulate blood clotting.

Protein deficiency leads to muscle weakness, anaemia, fluid retention, hair loss and increased risk of infection, so sufficient, high quality protein in the diet is essential for good health.

Mixing protein and carbohydrate in a meal

A general guide is that approximately 15-17% of the daily calories in a healthy diet should come from protein. Obviously the best way of achieving this is to combine carbohydrate and protein in a meal.

The richest and most easily absorbed forms of protein come from animal foods, not just meat or fish, but also eggs, milk and cheese or yoghurt. There are also protein rich plant foods although soya beans are the main plant source that contains all nine essential amino acids. Other plant foods do not have the same nutritional value as animal sources as they often only contain small amounts of some amino acids.

Mixing high quality protein with low GL carbohydrate food in a meal is the best and easiest way to ensure a healthy diet.

Choices can include things such as a sandwich made with wholegrain bread and lean ham or chicken, beans on wholegrain toast, wholemeal pasta with chicken, muesli with yoghurt or three bean chilli with wholemeal pitta bread.

Why fats are good

We seem to have developed a very difficult relationship with fat in the diet over recent years, actually eating far too much, especially of the wrong type, while thinking that we should have a totally fat free diet for health.

Neither extreme is correct.

We need a small amount of fat in our diet for good health. Fats are used for making cell membranes and prostaglandis, hormone like substances which regulate many of the bodily processes. The two main essential fatty acids (EFA's) are linoleic acid, which is an omega-6 fatty acid and linolenic acid, which is an omega-3 fatty acid.

Omega-6 fatty acids are found in vegetable oils, polyunsaturated margarine and products including these oils. They reduce LDL (bad) cholesterol but can also reduce HDL (good) cholesterol at very high intakes.

Omega-3 fatty acids are found in oily fish such as mackerel, salmon and sardines, dark leafy green vegetables such as spinach and kale, linseeds, pumpkin seeds, soya beans and walnuts. They are polyunsaturated fatty acids which include linolenic and its derivatives, which reduce the risk of blood clotting and therefore heart attacks and strokes.

Monounsaturated fatty acids such as olive oil, rapeseed oil, groundnut and hazelnut oils, nuts, seeds and avocados are liquid at room temperature and solidify when chilled. They reduce LDL cholesterol and maintain HDL cholesterol. They appear to reduce free radical damage which is associated with certain cancers, heart disease and rheumatoid arthritis. These are the fats that are thought to have the greatest health benefits.

A minimum of 15% fat, preferably unsaturated fatty acids is recommended in the diet. A totally fat free diet is not actually desirable, although you wouldn't think that when you look at all the low fat and fat free foods that are on the supermarket shelves. In fact, most processed low fat foods are actually full of sugar. If you look at two versions of the same food, one normal and one low fat, you should have a close look at the nutrition label. Although the reduction in fat percentage might not be that great, the sugar is quite often three or four times as much.

No matter what some diets would try to convince us, we need some fat in the diet so that we can obtain the fat-soluble vitamins A, D and E and make vitamin A from beta-carotene. We also need fat to absorb and transport fat-soluble vitamins in the body.

Why do we need fibre?

Fibre is an essential part of the diet for maintaining a healthy digestive system.

We obtain fibre from plant foods and although we generally have no problem in getting enough carbohydrate, protein and fat in our diets, most people fail to get enough fibre. Modern processed food and fast foods don't give us the levels of fibre that you find in a more traditional diet.

Foods high in fibre normally take longer to eat and can help you feel full because they slow down the digestion of the food. They also help slow the release of glucose and keep blood sugar levels more even. Feeling full and avoiding sugar spikes and sudden drops can help with weight control as you are less likely to feel hungry soon after a meal.

There are two types of fibre, soluble and insoluble.

Soluble fibre can be found in oats, rye, barley, fruits, vegetables and pulses. It helps slow the absorption of sugar and can help reduce the levels of blood sugar. It forms a gel-like mass during digestion which can bind cholesterol and therefore help reduce the levels of cholesterol in the blood.

As the term suggests, insoluble fibre doesn't dissolve and is not digested. It is found in the skins of vegetables and fruit, whole grain cereals and breads and brown rice. Combined with a sufficient fluid intake, it can help keep the gastro intestinal tract healthy and clean and help reduce the risk of constipation.

Vitamins and minerals

People have a tendency to think of vitamins and minerals as something that come in bottles of pills and have to be taken with food, but of course it is the food that gives us the vitamins and minerals we need. A healthy, well balanced diet should be more than enough to provide us with all the nutrients we need.

The body can produce a form of vitamin D in the skin with the help of sunlight and micro organisms in the intestinal tract produce vitamin K, but the vast majority of vitamins and minerals that we need have to be obtained from our food.

Why do we need vitamins?

Vitamins are essential for health, they help us process the carbohydrates, protein and fat in the food we eat. They help build cells, keep our skin healthy and protect us from free radicals and have a host of other benefits.

The vitamin content of food is at its highest when food is fresh. Fruits and vegetables build up the vitamin content as they mature to full ripeness and begin to lose their goodness soon after being picked, so ideally you would go out to the vegetable garden, pick your food and eat it. Unfortunately, that isn't possible for most people, so methods of storing and preparing food are very important.

Frozen foods are a good choice because they are normally harvested at peak freshness and then frozen, so when you take them from your freezer it is almost as good as picking them from your garden.

The two vitamin groups

Vitamins can be divided into two types, fat soluble and water soluble.

Our body treats them in different ways and it's important to take this into account when using them.

The fat soluble vitamins – A, D, E and K require fats for absorption and this means that they can be stored in the body and therefore can build up to possibly dangerous levels.

The water soluble vitamins – vitamin C and the B vitamins – do not store in the body, excess amounts are expelled from the body in urine. These are the vitamins that can be destroyed in the preparation of food, as they can dissolve if too much water is used in the cooking process. So rather than boiling the vegetables, steam or stir fry them, leaving texture rather than having them soggy and lacking their nutrients as well as their taste.

Vitamin A has an essential role in vision, especially night vision. It is also needed for bone growth, reproduction, healthy skin and for children's growth. The best natural sources of vitamin A are fish liver oils and it is very concentrated in animal liver. Other good sources are oily fish, egg yolk, butter and full fat milk.

The "B" vitamins, especially B_1, B_2 and B_3 are involved in releasing energy from the carbohydrates in the diet. The B vitamins are also involved in cell production and repair, and in maintaining a health immune system. Vitamin B_6, B12 and Folic acid are involved in the production of red blood cells.

The individual B vitamins have specific roles in the body.

Vitamin B_1, Thiamine helps maintain a health nervous and digestive system. Good sources are peas, spinach, beef, nuts, wholemeal bread and bran flakes

Vitamin B_2 Riboflavin works effectively with iron, vitamin B6 and folic acid and is essential in maintaining healthy skin, eyes and nerves. Good sources are Cottage cheese, asparagus, eggs, fish and meat.

Vitamin B_3 Niacin is essential for normal growth and healthy skin. It also helps to maintain a healthy nervous and digestive system. Good sources are oily fish, kidney beans, peanuts, and soya beans.

Vitamin B_5 Pantothenic acid is needed to make glucose and fatty acids from other metabolites in our bodies. It is also used in the manufacture of steroid hormones and brain chemicals and it maintains health skin, hair and immune system. Good sources are oily fish, sweet potatoes, mushrooms, lentils, beans and yoghurt.

Vitamin B_6 Pyridoxine is involved in protein and amino acid metabolism. It is needed for making red blood cells and new proteins and helps maintain a healthy immune system, which prevents us from getting ill. Good sources are potatoes, sweet potatoes, bananas, oily fish and chicken.

Vitamin B_{12} and Folic Acid are both involved with our red blood cell production in the bone marrow. They are also required for the division of cells and for making protein and DNA. Good sources are dairy products, offal, eggs and seafood.

Vitamin C, also known as ascorbic acid, is the least stable of the vitamins and very easily destroyed in cooking. It is essential in the formation of collagen, an important protein that strengthens bones and blood vessels, it also helps maintain good gum health. It is necessary for growth, tissue repair and healing wounds. It is an antioxidant and protects against infection by enabling white blood cells to break down bacteria and is involved in the production of red blood cells. It is also involved in the absorption of iron. Good sources are asparagus, kiwi fruit, citrus fruits, tomatoes and peppers.

Vitamin D helps our bodies absorb and use calcium and phosphorus, which are vital for building and maintaining strong and healthy bones. Good sources of vitamin D are dairy products (apart from low fat versions), oily fish, eggs and fortified margarine and breakfast cereals. We also produce a form of vitamin D in our skin with the help of sunlight, which is why it is important to spend some time outside in the sun, although it's not an excuse for lots of sunbathing.

Vitamin E is a powerful antioxidant. It prevents the oxidation of fatty acids in the cell membranes and protects our cells from damage. It also maintains healthy skin, heart and circulation, nerves, muscles and red blood cells. Good sources of vitamin E can be found in vegetable and seed oils, olive oil, oily fish, avocado, nuts, seeds, cereals, leafy green vegetables, wholemeal bread and egg yolk.

Vitamin K is needed for the formation of several of the proteins called "clotting factors" that regulate blood clotting. It is also needed for the formation of some proteins which are important for the maintenance of healthy bones and teeth. Good sources of vitamin K are from dark green leafy vegetables like broccoli, cabbage and spinach, potatoes, soya beans, liver, cheese and fruits. However, most of the vitamin K we need comes from the friendly bacteria, which live in our intestines.

Minerals

Like vitamins, minerals are essential for good health. They come from rocks and metal ores and enter the food chain by being taken up from the soil as plants grow. They are only needed in the body in tiny amounts, but they are vital.

Calcium is the main mineral in bones and teeth. It is also involved in blood clotting, nerve signals and muscle contraction. Absorption is helped by lactose, the sugar found in dairy products, and can be reduced by compounds found in vegetables such as spinach, beetroot, celery and parsley. Good sources of calcium are dairy products, almonds and tofu.

Magnesium also plays a vital role in the formation of bones and teeth as well as being involved in transmitting nerve signals and causing muscle contraction. It aids in the processing of fat and protein. Good sources are whole grains, spinach, bran flakes, red meat, nuts, beans and pulses.

Phosphorus is present in every cell of the body, but most of it is found in the bones and teeth. It helps the body use carbohydrates and fats and in the synthesis of protein for the growth, maintenance, and repair of cells and tissues. It is also part of ATP, a molecule the body uses to store energy. Good sources are whole grains - especially oats, dairy products, red meat, poultry and seafood.

Potassium is a very important mineral. It has various roles in metabolism and body functions and is essential for the proper function of all cells, tissues and organs. It helps in the regulation of the acid-alkali balance. It is involved in protein synthesis from amino acids and helps the body store blood sugar in the form of glycogen, the source of energy required by all muscles in the body. Good sources are whole grains, potatoes, avocadoes, red meat, dairy produce, oranges and broad beans

Sodium is vital for controlling the amount of water in the body and for maintaining the normal pH of blood, transmitting nerve signals and helping in muscular contraction. It is present in all foods in varying degrees and almost all processed foods have added sodium, so it is very easy to consume too much. A high concentration of sodium can lead to swelling, high blood pressure, difficulty in breathing and heart problems.

Sulphur plays a key role in the manufacture of amino acids and in the conversion of carbohydrates to a form that the body can use. It occurs in insulin, the hormone that regulates levels of blood sugar. Sulphur is also involved in manufacturing connective tissue, hair, skin and nails. It occurs naturally in all foods.

Chromium works with insulin, helping bind it to cell receptors and allowing blood sugar to move into the cell where it is needed for energy. Good sources are potatoes, broccoli, green beans, tomatoes, apples, bananas and grapes.

Copper plays a key role in several body functions including the production of pigment in skin, hair and eyes, the development of healthy bones, teeth and heart. It helps process iron in the body and with the formation of red blood cells and helps protect cells from chemical damage by working as an antioxident. Good sources are whole grains - especially barley, liver, crustaceans and nuts.

Fluoride is often added to tap water and is found mainly in the bones and teeth, helping increase bone density and reduce the risk of tooth decay. It can be obtained from water and any food that is prepared with water.

Iodine is needed for the metabolism of cells, converting food into energy. About 40% of iodine is stored in the thyroid gland and is used for the production of thyroid hormones which are required for normal body metabolism and growth. Good sources are sea food, lambs liver, eggs, peanuts, wholemeal bread, cheddar cheese, green peppers, milk, cream, lamb, raisins.

Iron is an essential mineral in all cells of the body, even though it is only needed in minute amounts. It is needed to make haemoglobin, the oxygen carrying protein found in red blood cells and myoglobin, a protein found in muscle cells. It is involved in the release of energy from glucose and fatty acids in the intestine. Good sources are red meat, offal, poultry, spinach, dried fruit, egg yolks, tuna, prawns and pulses.

Selenium is an antioxidant and as such can play a role in preventing cell damage from free radicals. It is vital for a healthy immune system and thyroid gland and possibly can protect against cancer. Good sources are shellfish, especially oysters, brown rice, wheat germ, wholemeal bread and Brazil nuts.

Zinc is essential for the breakdown of carbohydrates, protein and fats. It is needed for the immune system and plays a role in cell division, cell growth and wound healing. Zinc is also needed for the senses of smell and taste and is essential for sexual maturation, fertility and reproduction. Good sources are oysters, dairy products, red meat, eggs, Brazil nuts, haricot beans and soya beans.

Should you take vitamin and mineral supplements

The ideal life style is to obtain the required vitamins and minerals from a healthy, balanced diet, but there are times when supplementation can help. This can be because the diet is restricted, such as a vegetarian or vegan diet, or at certain times in life, such as pregnancy or menopause, or with certain lifestyles such as smoking or being on a diet that restricts the amount of food eaten. Supplements can also be useful at certain times of the year, such as during the winter.

Although the advice is that you should be able to get enough of all the vitamins and minerals that you need in a well balanced, healthy diet, the fact is that the very way some of our food is produced reduces the nutritional value of it before it even reaches the kitchen.

You can also reduce the goodness of the food in the cooking process – by boiling vegetables for too long, or keeping fresh food too long before using it. The nutritional value of fresh fruit and vegetables begins to reduce as soon as it is harvested, so by the time it is shipped half way around the world, packaged, taken to the supermarket, waits on the shelves for you to buy it and then taken home and used a few days later, a lot of the goodness is already gone.

So although you should aim to get all the vitamins and minerals from a healthy diet, it can sometimes be very difficult.

If you are using a supplement, it's best to choose a good quality multi vitamin and mineral tablet because vitamins and minerals interact with each other, either competing with each other for absorption or helping the effectiveness of one another. This means that taking supplements of single vitamins or minerals can actually lead to deficiencies and imbalances. Although we think of supplements as 'all good' you can actually have an overdose of some vitamins, so it's important to take some advice before deciding to superdose yourself.

Too much vitamin A can lead to liver damage and blurred vision, too much vitamin D can lead to a build up of calcium deposits.

So choose a good quality multi vitamin and check with a medical professional before adding too many supplements to your daily routine, especially if you are taking other medication.

Finally...

Our bodies are designed to be finely tuned and although they can take a lot of punishment and still keep us functioning, it's worth trying to keep the whole system balanced.

There is so much information about food, especially about how to eat less of it, and so many of the diets are based around restricting certain food groups that it's very difficult to work out what exactly is a good, healthy diet.

Understanding what food actually does for the body, instead of just seeing it as the enemy, is the first step in the journey to having that magical healthy, balanced diet. And that is the first step in the journey to a healthy, well balanced body.

Your body is a temple – make sure it's not one of the Roman Ruins!

About the Author

Marianne Duvall's passion in life is showing people how to make it easy to live a healthier life through nutrition and fitness – making small changes in everyday life that can make big changes in health and wellbeing.

She has studied how to rebalance modern life to allow space for good nutrition and activity as part of everyday life rather than an expensive and time consuming extra.

She believes that healthy living should be how we live, part of everyday life rather than an afterthought. Something so natural that we don't even think about it, we just do it.

She has developed her ideas over the years working with those living with chronic illnesses such as M.E./CFS, fibromyalgia or diabetes, developing plans that help people live successfully with these illnesses.

Her motto is 'Live Life'